Allergies

MW00961003

Ways to help increase the safety and awareness of food allergies.

by Stacey Stratton
Copyright © 2016
All rights reserved
Images © www.bigstock.com

About the Author: Stacey Stratton has an M.A. in Education and over 8 years experience working in the Special Education field. Her experience not only includes educating others, but being an advocate for those who have any type of special need. She's the founder of the AllergyFreeZone.com and has worked as the Publications Manager for the Food Allergy & Anaphylaxis Connection Team (FAACT). Stacey has also written numerous articles and blog posts about food allergies.

Disclaimer: The content posted in this book is not intended and should not replace professional medical information or advice. Discuss all questions of a medical nature with your doctor or allergist.

This book is designed to be a discussion guide when working with your allergist and school. Please note: School policies and procedures, along with laws and regulations may differ in your specific area.

Note: EpiPen® and Benadryl® are referenced in the book and are registered trademarks.

Dedications and Acknowledgements

This book is dedicated to YOU. I hope it will give you guidance in working with your school, so together you can implement ways to increase your child's safety. The changes you make in your schools and communities will greatly affect the lives of all families who have children with food allergies. THANK YOU for all that YOU do!

"Thank You" to organizations like the Food Allergy & Anaphylaxis Connection Team (FAACT), Food Allergy Research & Education (FARE), Kids With Food Allergies (KFA), and many other organizations that are out there educating and advocating.

And "Thank You" to my sister Denise for all your help and support throughout the years.

Be sure to visit:
www.allergyfreezone.com
www.facebook.com/allergyfreezone
www.twitter.com/allergyfreezone
www.pinterest.com/allergyfreezone

Peanut & Nut Allergies?
www.facebook.com/peanutfreezone

Introduction

It can be difficult trying to find the right questions to ask, and so many times we think of things to say.... after a meeting is over. This book is meant to guide you, prepare you, and help you discover different topics to discuss with your child's school.

The Allergy Free Zone has helpful TIPs, including free downloads and resources that you can share with your child's school. We also have awareness products like stickers, signs, tattoos, and bags to help inform and remind others of your child's food allergy.

FREE PRINTABLES
Be sure to get your two free printables
"Tips for Parents" and "Tips for Teachers" at:
www.allergyfreezone.com

It's very easy to feel like you're all alone. No one really understands what you're going through like someone who's going through the same thing. Before school starts, ask the school if they can put you in contact with other parents who have children with food allergies. You might also want to consider finding a food allergy support group, playgroup, or even start one of your own. You can find links to support groups in the resource section of this book.

For encouragement, support, and food allergy TIPs...
Visit: www.facebook.com/allergyfreezone

Table of Contents

Chapter 1

Getting Prepared

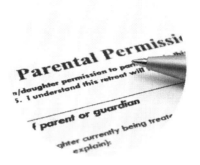

Whether your child is starting kindergarten or entering a new school building, anticipating this event in your child's life can seem scary. Contacting the school as soon as possible will give everyone time to prepare for your child's first day.

If this is the first time you've had a child in this particular school, try to visit during a school day and see how things operate. Call ahead and see if there's a convenient time you can schedule a visit. Introduce yourself to the principal and office staff, and let them know about your child's food allergy.

Have them introduce you to the school nurse. Be sure to find out if the nurse is assigned to different schools or will be in your child's school everyday. If they don't have a full-time nurse, do they have a health aide or someone trained in handling an allergic reaction?

Troubleshooting Areas

When walking around the school, pay attention to things like vending machines, cafeteria menu, table locations, and restroom locations (for hand washing). What is the layout of the classroom and where are the lockers/cubbies located? Is there a sink in the classroom? Bring a notebook and write down any questions or concerns you may have, so you can later discuss them.

Find out if they have any other students with food allergies and what precautions are currently being made for them. Ask if they can put you in contact with the parents of the children who have food allergies. These parents could become a great support for you and help ease any anxiety you may be experiencing.

Depending on privacy issues, they might not be able to give you that information. If this is an issue, ask if they would be willing to pass along your contact information to the parents.

Scheduling a Team Meeting

Discuss having a team meeting with the principal, nurse, and all other staff members who will play a vital role in your child's safety. This may include the cafeteria supervisor, head custodian, teachers, bus driver, etc.

Find out how and when the staff members receive training on food allergy safety and on administering epinephrine. Do they understand life-threatening allergies, or will you need to direct them to educational materials and resources? Ask the school if there's anything you can help provide.

Discuss when will be the best time to have the meeting. If you have the meeting before summer break, they might need to retrain everyone at the beginning of the school year. But, it might be helpful to give them heads-up, and allow them to learn more about food allergies over the summer.

At the end of summer, teachers and staff usually start getting ready a week or two before students arrive. This might be an ideal time to meet with them, as they're not preoccupied yet with lesson plans and class needs.

School forms

Find out what forms you'll need for your child. Do they have downloadable forms from the school's website or will you pick them up in the school office? Do they have a specific Food Allergy Action Plan form that they use or will you need to provide one? You can find links to free allergy action plans in our resource section. If the school has their own form, use their form so it complies with their procedures and doesn't get mistaken for other documentation.

Make sure you gather all the forms you'll need to take to the doctor/allergist, and any other forms or information they'll require from you before the beginning of the school year. Fill out the forms completely and don't hesitate to have them explain anything you don't understand. Consider adding allergy alert stickers to draw attention to your child's paperwork. You can find allergy alert stickers at www.allergyfreezone.com.

Make an appointment with your child's allergist. Make sure you also factor in a busy schedule, especially the closer it gets to the end of summer. Many people are often rushing right before or during the first week of school to get their medical forms filled out.

If your child qualifies for a 504 or IEP, the school may require extra documentation. You can find out more about 504s and IEPs in our resource section.

Asking Questions

Think about different questions you'll want to ask the allergist and write down topics you'll want to discuss, so you won't forget.

At the appointment - don't be afraid to bring up any questions you may have. Request documentation of the food allergy, prescriptions, and any other materials you may need to give the school. Have the allergist fill out your child's allergy action plan and explain everything in it to you.

Ask the allergist to clearly state the details of your child's food allergy, along with the precautions that need to be taken, and the reasons why. Is there any additional information the allergist feels the staff will need to know?

If your child has asthma, discuss if they should use an epinephrine auto-injector if they're unsure if your child is having an asthma attack or allergic reaction. Also discuss with your allergist what will happen if someone mistakenly uses the epinephrine when it's not truly needed.

Are there any risks or reasons they should use caution? Be sure to document this information and discuss it with the team members at the meeting.

Before leaving, make sure you understand everything that was discussed. Try repeating everything back to the allergist to make sure you heard everything correctly (this includes going over how to use the epinephrine auto-injector).

Keeping Records

Keep everything stored in a binder or other organized method so you'll know where to quickly find them.

Make copies of all paperwork you supply to the school. They can easily misplace forms when they have so much paperwork at the beginning of the school year. You can save yourself the trouble of having to get the forms filled out again if the school needs another copy, and you'll have extra copies for your records.

If your child is older, consider having them attend the meeting with you. This will be an excellent opportunity for the staff to get to know your child, and will help teach advocacy skills to your child.

CHECKLIST

- ✓ Call the school to introduce yourself to the principal & nurse
- ✓ Visit the school to see the environment and meet any available staff
- ✓ Bring a notebook to list all questions and concerns
- ✓ Can you contact the other parents who have children with allergies?
- ✓ Pick up all school forms
- ✓ Make appointment with allergist
- ✓ Discuss all questions, concerns, and go over forms with allergist
- ✓ Keep records and notes – document everything
- ✓ Make copies of all paperwork before giving to the school

NOTES

Chapter 2

The Team Meeting

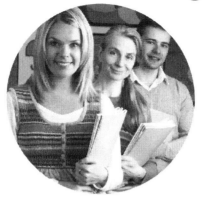

If you haven't done so already, find out when you can have a team meeting to introduce yourself to the staff and discuss your child's needs. This meeting can help bring everyone together to discuss your child's food allergy, and develop safety procedures for creating a safer environment.

The meeting may include the principal or administrative representative, nurse, cafeteria supervisor, classroom teachers and specialists, counselors, gym teacher, custodian, bus driver, attendants/aides, and coaches or leaders of after-school activities. Anyone who'll be in direct contact with your child should be encouraged to attend.

Discussing Plans

At the meeting, review the allergy action plan that was developed with your child's allergist. Let them know the key points that were discussed with the allergist and give them copies of the documentation. If they use an IHCP (Individual Health Care Plan), the team might also discuss and complete this paperwork at the meeting.

Go over the warning signs of an allergic reaction and steps to take in an emergency. Discuss how and where the epinephrine will be stored and who will be trained to administer it in an emergency. This will be discussed further in Chapter 3.

Find out when you should bring your child's epinephrine and other medications, so they're placed in the proper locations before the first day of school. Often, the first several days are the most chaotic and therefore could pose a higher risk for a reaction to occur when staff is overwhelmed with new faces and procedures.

Make sure everyone knows that time is critical and they should not hesitate if they think there's an emergency. If they choose to wait and see....it could cost your child their life!

504

Discuss setting up a 504 meeting and having a 504 plan in place for your child. 504s are encouraged because it's a written plan of how the school will address the individual needs of your child, including being able to participate safely and equally with their peers during the school day.

Discuss Stories

Share any stories of what you experienced when your child had a reaction. Bring any pictures of what a reaction may look like or has looked like on your child. This can help them understand certain things they need to watch for in your child.

Discuss stories of other children who have had reactions at school. This is especially important if they don't seem to understand the seriousness of the allergy. Actual articles would be good to print out and share. We have provided several article links in Chapter 10.

Training

If you feel comfortable, offer to help the school with any training or educational materials you may have on allergies. Find out how and when they'll train their staff, and if they'll repeat the training throughout the year.

If they are new to food allergies, encourage them to contact a local food allergy support group, as some will gladly assist the school. There are also some websites that have training provided online. More information on this is provided in our resource section.

Important topics staff members will need to learn about: Recognizing the signs and symptoms of an allergic reaction, epinephrine auto-injector administration, label reading and the different names used for the allergen, proper cleaning of the allergen from surfaces, and avoiding cross-contact.

The school should consider having drills on responding to an anaphylactic emergency, throughout the school year. This can be a very scary situation for everyone involved and they must not have ANY doubt on what they need to do to help the child.

Substitutes

How will they handle different substitutes in the building to make sure they're aware and prepared to handle an emergency? Will the substitute be able to be trained before the school day starts?

Discuss if the person scheduling the substitutes can check if they're comfortable with their assignment when scheduling. It would be helpful to have the same sub if possible, that way they're familiar with your child and their allergy action plan.

Writing Letters

Find out who will write the letters to the other parents to let them know about your child's allergy. Depending on the area that you live, can the materials be translated in French and Spanish for parents that are unable to read English?

Encourage them to have a letter prepared to send home on the first day of school. Let the parents know there's a life-threatening food allergy in their child's classroom, and what precautions will need to be taken. Parents are accustomed to reviewing many papers the first few days of school and this is critical information for them to know immediately.

Snacks/Lunches

Find out if it's possible to have a "no food" policy in the classroom. If food is allowed, can there be a policy of "no food" for the first couple weeks until all allergies are known & explained?

Discuss hand washing for your child and their classmates, before/after lunch and snacks. Is it possible to have the students wash their hands at the start of the day in case they had peanut butter or other allergens before arriving at school?

Discuss how the students' packed lunches are stored. Will your child be able to keep their lunch separated and carry it with them to the cafeteria? Do they have an area in the lunchroom that will be safe for your child to eat?

Do they have Peanut Free Zone Signs or Allergy Alert Signs for the area? If not, find out if the signs are something you can provide or if the school will purchase or make them. There are several different signs available at: www.allergyfreezone.com.

Other Discussion Topics

Different fundraising methods are something schools often use. Discuss the possibility of refraining from having a bake sale or selling candy as fundraising events. See if they can look into non-food ways to raise money, so your child can participate too.

Staff meetings are often held in the library and food is sometimes provided. Request that these types of meetings or activities aren't held in a room that your child will be using. If an event that involves food would happen to occur in the room, discuss making sure the area is properly cleaned before your child arrives.

Find out if there will be teaching assistants/aides or class helpers to help out in the classroom or during certain activities like lunch and recess.

Do they have policies in place for bullying or teasing a child because of their food allergy, and what are the consequences?

Communication Tips

You may get some resistance at the meeting. Don't go in as the "know-it-all". If you start demanding certain things are done, it might put them more on the defense and could make them less likely to offer any suggestions.

In some situations it will be helpful to brainstorm with them, or encourage them towards an idea. You might say, "It would be very helpful if_____. Do you know of any way it could possibly be accomplished?" Even if you already have an idea of how it could be done, let them help figure out a solution. They might have a better idea than what you originally thought. Plus, if they're the ones who think of it, they might take more ownership in making sure it gets done.

In the book *The 7 Habits of Highly Effective Teens* by Stephen Covey, Step 5 is "Seek first to understand, then be understood." If you really think about it, that's powerful advice! Really listen to what they're saying and try to figure out what is causing them to respond that way. This is especially important if someone is being very defensive.

Find out if any of them have children. If they do, try to put them in your shoes. Share your heart and let them know how you are truly feeling as a parent.

Don't be afraid that you're being overdramatic. If your child has a life-threating food allergy..... exposure can be fatal. If you get emotional, don't feel foolish or regretful of how you acted. It's your child's life - you have every right to get emotional.

Don't assume everyone understands. Some people don't want to look foolish and they may just nod their head when they really have no clue. Be sure to ask questions that need an actual response.

When you're talking to them, you should be able to tell when someone finally "gets it". Some won't, and you WILL have to repeat this information throughout the school year. Even if they do "get it"....you WILL have to repeat this information throughout the school year.

Protecting your child from exposure to the allergen is vital. Ask and discuss if they know any other ways they can help reduce the risk of exposure.

Thank them during the meeting, but also thank them after the meeting. Sending team members a handwritten note is a nice way to express how much you appreciate their help in keeping your child safe. It can also be a great reminder of your child's food allergy and safety needs.

CHECKLIST

- ✓ Schedule the meeting
- ✓ Review allergy action plan and other documentation from allergist
- ✓ Go over any signs and symptoms of a past reaction
- ✓ Discuss stories of other children if appropriate
- ✓ Discuss 504 plans, IHCP and other school plans
- ✓ Offer material and training suggestions if needed
- ✓ Who will inform other parents of the allergy?
- ✓ Who will train staff?
- ✓ "No food" policy in classroom?
- ✓ Safely storing and eating lunch
- ✓ Cleaning allergen from areas the child will use
- ✓ The policies and consequences for bullying/teasing
- ✓ Using aides and helpers to help watch over child
- ✓ Training and informing substitutes
- ✓ Help them brainstorm in the meeting
- ✓ Don't assume everyone understands
- ✓ Send a handwritten "Thank You" to team members

NOTES

Chapter 3

The School Nurse

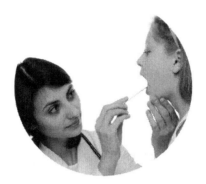

Introduce your child to the nurse as soon as possible. You'll want both your child and the nurse to have time to meet and develop a relationship. This might also help your child feel more comfortable about starting school.

The nurse has such an important job, and unfortunately with school budgets, sometimes having a nurse in each school is impossible. They might only be able to come to the school on certain days of the week. If there isn't a full-time nurse, find out who will be there to handle a medical emergency in their absence.

You might need to frequently communicate with the nurse to make sure all the paperwork is in place before the first day of school. This will include providing forms from the child's doctor/allergist, along with any required medical forms from the school.

Current Information

The school will always need to have a current contact number to reach you in an emergency. A cell phone that's always with you is a must. List any other numbers where you can be contacted, along with the numbers of any other family members that can be notified. Also, make sure they always have the current information on your child's allergist and doctor.

Make sure your child's medication is labeled, and keep a record of the expiration dates to know when they need to be replaced. This may include the epinephrine auto-injectors (EpiPen®, etc.), Benadryl®, and any other medications prescribed by the doctor/allergist.

TIP: When you're purchasing your epinephrine auto-injectors, make sure you look at the date so you don't accidentally get one with a short expiration date. Smaller pharmacies may be able to get one shipped to you directly from the manufacturer. If you have to self-pay, call around to different pharmacies – sometimes you can find them for a lower price. Also, consider calling the manufacturer and asking if they have a coupon available for those who self-pay for medication.

Where will your child's medication be located? Minutes matter during a severe reaction, and your child's medication should not be stored in a locked area that's far away from them. Make sure you understand and are comfortable with where the medication will be located. This is also something you should discuss and have documented by your allergist before the team meeting.

If your child states they're not feeling well and needs to see the nurse, they should never go to the nurse alone. Make sure someone always accompanies them or the nurse is called to their location immediately.

Find out how the nurse is notified of an emergency. The nurse should always have a direct line of communication available at all times. If the nurse isn't there full-time, what's the protocol? If there's a substitute nurse, how will they be informed of your child's allergy and action plan?

Staff Training

Ask about staff training. Will they train all staff members and how many times will they receive training throughout the year? Will they have drills to practice what to do in an anaphylactic emergency? Will the nurse provide info and training to substitute teachers, cafeteria workers, etc.?

Nurses should help provide materials to teach about allergy awareness and provide copies of the allergy action plan to everyone that's involved in your child's safety. They should also consider providing a script to call 911, that's placed by all the school phones.

Find out if they've ever had to administer an epinephrine auto-injector and how they handled the emergency. Make sure there's also a plan of who will go to the hospital and stay with your child until a family member arrives.

The school needs to have a plan in place that is understood and rehearsed by everyone, so they'll know exactly what they need to do in an emergency.

CHECKLIST

- ✓ Introduce yourself and your child – start building a relationship
- ✓ Make sure all forms and paperwork are filled out properly
- ✓ Label medication and record expiration dates
- ✓ Make sure all contact numbers and information is current
- ✓ Discuss what they will do in emergency situations
- ✓ Discuss training staff and substitutes
- ✓ If the nurse isn't there full-time, who handles everything?

NOTES

Chapter 4

Playgrounds and Recess

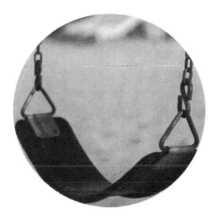

Playgrounds can be a higher-risk area for a child with a peanut allergy. Often times, children attend recess right after lunch. If they haven't washed their hands, they could possibly contaminate the equipment with the allergen.

This is also a time when children might carry out food from lunch or eat candy that was hidden in their pockets. An adult should watch that children don't try to eat food or candy on the playground. Is there a school policy that no food is allowed on the playground?

Monitors

Make sure your child has a "go-to face"...and it's the same person every day. If possible, a person who is specifically assigned to watch your child would be best. General playground monitors have to watch everything, and sometimes recess can be chaos. There's a lot of noise (kids yelling and screaming) and a child having a reaction could be overlooked. The monitor will need to easily recognize your child and should watch them from the moment they walk out the doors, to the time they walk back in.

This adult must be familiar with the allergy action plan, and be trained in administering an epinephrine auto-injector. Request that your child's epinephrine and allergy action plan are easily accessible, and discuss how that can be made possible.

They need to have some form of communication like a cell phone or walkie-talkie, so they can call for help immediately if there's any type of emergency. The monitor must take all complaints and comments from your child seriously.

They also need to listen for any bullying or teasing towards your child because of their allergy. If your child feels threatened in any way, encourage them to get in sight of the monitor so they can feel more protected. It's best if they can even get somewhere that the monitor can hear what's going on in the situation. Sometimes monitors can't do anything if they haven't seen or heard the "bullying".

Have a Buddy

When a child is having an allergic reaction, they may not be able to communicate what's happening to them. The child should have at least one "buddy" that they're partnered up with on the playground. Make sure the buddy knows they need to immediately seek help if they're concerned how their friend looks or acts.

Have a plan for when the monitor is absent, and make sure your child can easily identify and feels comfortable with the fill-in monitor. Make sure the fill-in monitor has been properly trained.

Since playground equipment is often used during non-school hours, a visual inspection for all safety issues should be conducted before the children start playing each day. Ask if they can also look for and clean up any wrappers or food that may have been left behind.

CHECKLIST

✓ Have a monitor watching your child

✓ Discuss playground rules about eating food

✓ Monitor needs quick access to epinephrine and the allergy action plan

✓ Monitor must be trained in what to do in an anaphylactic emergency

✓ Monitor needs to have a form of communication instantly accessible

✓ Watch for bullying and teasing

✓ Assign a buddy to watch for any changes

✓ Check area for contamination

NOTES

Chapter 5

Field Trips

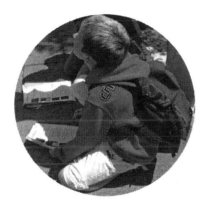

The thought of your child having a food allergy and attending a field trip can be very scary. At the beginning of the year, discuss avoiding high-risk places like sporting events, restaurants, and food or candy factory tours. Make sure the school and teacher both know that you'll need to be notified as soon as possible of any scheduled field trips or activities involving food.

Chaperones

Depending on your work schedule or other daily responsibilities, see if it's possible to go chaperone the activity. If you're unable to attend the field trip, see if a family member or friend (that understands food allergies) is willing to chaperone. Grandparents, aunts, etc., make great field trip attendees.

Sometimes it will be another classroom parent that is willing to watch over your child. Make sure they're not assigned to supervise an entire group, which could easily distract them from their purpose. Watching to keep your child safe should be their main duty on the field trip.

The person watching over your child's safety will always need to be with your child and have the medicine easily accessible. This person must understand the allergy action plan and know what to do in an emergency. They must also understand that they need to take all complaints and comments about food allergies seriously.

During the field trip, a cell phone or other form of communication must be available to quickly contact others in an emergency. All emergency information (address of facility, location of hospital, etc.) and medical forms must also be readily available.

Find out what type of transportation they'll take – bus, van, walking? If they're taking a bus or van, also look at Chapter 7 for transportation safety.

Lunches and Food

Discuss the plans for lunch and/or snacks, and if food will be brought or purchased. See if the teacher can send out a letter asking other parents to refrain from sending in any items that contain the allergen.

Find out how the students will be able to clean their hands before and after eating. If any students handle the allergen, they should wash their hands to avoid spreading the allergen during the field trip.

If the students bring snacks or their lunch, have them keep your child's lunch separated. Many kids will pack easy items for a field trip, like peanut butter & jelly sandwiches. Someone should also watch that the students aren't getting into their lunches before or after the designated time.

Contact Facility

Contact the facility directly to discuss your child's food allergy and the safety of the environment. Ask the facility if it's possible to have one of the tables thoroughly cleaned and reserved for your child's use.

Your child could also use a placemat, multiple napkins, or rip open their lunch bag to use as a barrier to help protect placing food directly on the table.

Many times, the locations they visit will pass out treats or baked goods. I highly recommend teaching your child beforehand to not accept the item and give a standard reply like, "No thank you, I have a food allergy".

Also, find out the activities they'll be doing on their field trip. Make sure they won't be exposed to the allergen if feeding animals or making crafts.

Consider having them wear a temporary tattoo, zipper pull, or other item to help bring attention and remind others of the allergy. Make sure their lunch bag and beverages are clearly marked with a sticker or other method. You can find stickers, tattoos and zipper pulls at www.allergyfreezone.com.

If you don't feel comfortable about the place, the activities, or how your child will be chaperoned... Don't be afraid to speak up! If you feel it's best that your child skips the trip, consider taking them somewhere else and having a special day of your own.

CHECKLIST

- ✓ Contact the facility directly to find out more about the safety of the environment and activities
- ✓ Will the students have access to food?
- ✓ Will the students pack or purchase lunch or snacks?
- ✓ Will the eating area be cleaned and have safe area for your child?
- ✓ Can students clean their hands before and after eating?
- ✓ How will they get to the location?
- ✓ Who will be in charge of watching over your child?
- ✓ Who will know how to administer the epinephrine auto-injector?
- ✓ Who will carry the allergy action plan, epinephrine auto-injector and other medical info?
- ✓ Phone number to reach the field trip (teacher) if needed?
- ✓ If your child has a cell phone, can they take it?
- ✓ Use awareness items to help inform/remind others of the allergy.

NOTES

Chapter 6

The Cafeteria

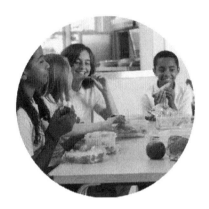

All cafeteria workers need to know about the food allergy and be able to easily recognize your child. Make sure your child is introduced to them at the beginning of the year, especially to those who will have direct contact on a daily basis. They should have a photo of your child, along with their allergy information placed in the supervisor's office or somewhere they can view it often throughout the year.

Checking Products

The supervisor of the cafeteria needs to check the products before purchasing and read the labels EVERY time it's purchased, along with the manufacturing information. Products and manufacturing often change! They also need to know all the other ingredient names that contain the allergen. Make sure they know they can easily print out label reading and ingredient information sheets (you can find info in our resource section).

Food service companies may switch food items without informing the school. Make sure companies know specific items they're not allowed to use as substitutes. If possible, someone in the cafeteria should check all the products as soon as they arrive so they can immediately address any issues and send back any items.

The FDA has requirements for listing the eight major food allergens on labels, but how the product is manufactured is voluntary information and may or may not be provided from the companies. Be sure to visit www.fda.gov for more information on Food Allergen Labeling.

Phone numbers and contact information for the food companies need to be stored and called whenever there's a question about the safety of a product.

ALL cafeteria workers should be trained in properly reading labels, especially if the manager or supervisor has to leave for an extended period of time. It would be beneficial to have a book with all the food allergy safety procedures in one place, so someone could easily follow it if they had to temporarily fill the position.

Will the nurse provide the medical training to the cafeteria workers? Can they have drills and role-play scenarios to help the workers prepare for different situations? Will someone compile a folder with safety procedures and review information with lunchroom subs? These are all great questions you can ask.

Cooks, Servers and Cashiers

ALL cooks and servers need to understand about cross-contact and how to avoid it when preparing and serving the food. This includes making sure they're not using the same rag and bucket to clean surfaces that may have been contaminated.

Servers need to know about the child's food allergy to help ensure the allergen is not accidentally given to the child. They must also make sure the serving utensils are ONLY used for that specific item. They should use clean non-latex gloves before handling the child's food.

Cashiers also need to watch the child doesn't accidentally try to purchase an "unsafe" item, including any packaged snacks. Some schools have a computer system that reminds the cashier about the child's allergy and instantly notifies them if they're accidentally trying to purchase something containing the allergen.

One company that provides this type of system is AllerSchool. Unfortunately, this type of equipment might be impossible for some schools to purchase due to budget constraints.

If your school keeps track of money through a keypad where students enter their number, ask if a staff member can enter the number for your child. This can help avoid exposure to possible allergens that may have contaminated the keypad.

Find out if it's possible to print out monthly lunch menus that have the allergens listed on the menu. Some schools also provide a list on their website stating all their food items and their allergens. If the ingredients or manufacturing changes - everyone must be informed of the changes immediately.

Sometimes schools may have a special lunch like "pizza day" where pizzas are brought in from a local shop. Ask to receive advanced notice of any special lunches, so you can pack your child something special in their lunch or make a dinner they'll look forward to that evening.

If you want to ensure the safety of what your child will be served for lunch, send it from home. Even if the school says the lunches are safe – it's safer (and usually healthier) to pack your child's lunch. If you want your child to have school beverages, ask how your child can safely get it. Can they be first in line or can a staff member get the item for them?

Develop a plan for what will happen if your child forgets their lunch or money. As soon as it's known that the lunch has been forgotten, have the school call you immediately. At that time, you can decide what can be done to make sure your child is provided with a safe lunch. Discuss the back-up lunch options that the school provides to make sure it's not something your child can't have, like a peanut butter sandwich. One plan might be to have them give your child some of their safe snacks and a safe school beverage.

Custodians and Lunch Aides

Custodians and lunch aides should be able to easily recognize your child and have knowledge of their food allergy.

Lunch aids should carry around pictures of the students with food allergies (especially during the first few weeks) to make sure they know who is allergic to what, and where they sit. They must know the exact steps of what they will need to do in an emergency.

Lunch aides should help watch that no food, drinks, or utensils are shared. They need to pay attention to any type of bullying, teasing or comments from other students.

Lunch aides also need to watch for any changes in your child and take all complaints seriously. If your child is feeling any type of illness, it's important that they don't walk to the nurse or bathroom alone.

Peanut Free and Other Allergen Free Zones

Find out if they will they designate a special table for a Peanut Free Zone or other Allergen-Free area where your child can safely sit at lunch.

Custodians need to clean the table before each use by using a disposable rag (or a clean rag used for that area only), hot water, and an approved cleaning solution to remove any traces of the allergen. A clean bucket should be clearly labeled and used only for that table. There should be a trash can for the child's use, that isn't used by the rest of the students.

Once the table has been properly cleaned, a sign can be placed on the table to confirm and assure others that the table is clean and ready for use. Your child can also eat out of their lunch box, place their lunch on a napkin, or tear a paper lunch bag open to make a placemat.

The table should be located in an area that is still part of the lunchroom. This could be the corner table or a table placed on the stage. Your child should NEVER feel isolated, embarrassed or made to eat alone!

They can have lunch friends sit with them (which is HIGHLY encouraged so they aren't alone) as long as their lunches are free from the allergen. Ask the teacher if they can be in charge of assigning weekly friends to sit with your child. They can easily go alphabetically down the class roster and give the parents notice of what day their child needs to pack a "safe" lunch. If the classmate forgets to pack a safe lunch, the classmate will just sit at the regular table instead.

If the cafeteria is also a gym, make sure the floor is properly cleaned before gym class starts. Custodians should thoroughly clean all tables and chairs before putting them away.

Other Areas of Concern

Drinking fountains should also be cleaned frequently, although use of them for your child is not encouraged. Instead, you may want to have your child use a water bottle that is marked for their use only.

Vending machines can be a hazard, as many kids get items at the end of their lunch period and bring them out of the cafeteria. See if the school can substitute allergen items (like peanut butter cups) with safer and healthier choices. Ask them about the possibility of limiting access to vending machines to after-school only.

CHECKLIST

✓ Recognizing your child and knowing about their allergy

✓ Training on label reading and cross-contamination

✓ Contacting companies for product questions

✓ Following food safety rules with serving utensils and non-latex gloves

✓ Having a folder with safety procedures and reviewing with subs

✓ Watching items containing the allergen aren't purchased

✓ Having a plan for an alternative lunch if needed

✓ Knowing what to do in an emergency

✓ Watching for bullying, food sharing, and any changes in your child

✓ Taking all complaints seriously

✓ Properly cleaning all surfaces - tables, floors, chairs, etc.

✓ Designating a specific area in the lunchroom free of the allergen

✓ Making sure child isn't isolated, embarrassed, or made to eat alone

NOTES

Chapter 7

Using School Transportation

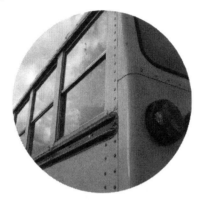

If you plan on having your child ride the bus to and from school, ask the school about scheduling a meeting with the bus driver assigned to your route. Make sure the allergy action plan has been reviewed with the driver and all necessary paperwork has been filled out before the first day.

Find out their rules for eating on the bus and bullying/teasing. How are rules enforced and violations handled? Will these rules be communicated and visibly posted on the bus?

An Assigned Seat

Find out if your child can have an assigned seat and how often it will be cleaned. Assigned seating is highly recommended and your child should sit in the first two seats so the bus driver can keep a close eye on them.

Morning can be a concerning time because many children are finishing breakfast right before the bus arrives. If they still have the allergen on their hands, contaminating areas like the handrails and seat backs is possible.

As your child gets older and comfort level increases, they can move back a bit. But for the early years, consider having them stay up front with a neighborhood friend sitting with them. The friend should understand food allergy safety, so they'll know how to help prevent exposure and when to call for help.

It's often loud on the bus and can be difficult for the driver to hear what's going on behind them. By having a friend or advocate sit by your child (preferably a neighbor who gets on and off around the same time) they can help watch for any changes and quickly get the driver's attention if needed.

A couple other reasons your child should sit up front: A lot of kids sneak food on the bus - they raid their lunch boxes on the way to school because they didn't eat breakfast, or they finish off their lunch on the way home. It's difficult to impossible for the bus driver to see what's going on in the back of the bus. If your child were to start having a reaction, the bus driver can possibly see and reach them quicker if they're in close proximity.

Do they have a policy for a child wearing or carrying an epinephrine auto-injector? You might be asked to supply one to the bus driver, but if they're leaving it on the bus, it could be subject to fluctuating temperatures and become ruined.

Who will train the bus driver on recognizing and responding to an allergic reaction? If there's a medical emergency on the bus, the bus driver will need a plan on how to respond if it happens while they're driving. The driver should always have emergency numbers instantly accessible and know the quickest route to a medical facility.

Different Buses and Drivers

Find out how they'll inform a substitute bus driver about your child's allergy and action plan, and who'll provide the medical training for substitute bus drivers. Also, ask if your child will have more than one bus driver (a different one for morning and afternoon), which is often common for kindergarten.

You will also want to know the route of the bus and how long your child will be on it. Is your house one of the first stops or one of the last? Will your child ride multiple buses? Some schools transport children from one school and then they get on another bus to their destination.

Will the bus also be used for field trips or after-school events? Find out if they can clean the bus after these types of events, where students may have been eating on it.

On the first day of school, you'll want to introduce your child to the bus driver. Make sure your child knows what seat is assigned to them. Then, take a moment to watch them enjoy the bus they've probably been looking forward to riding for years!

If you don't feel comfortable with the busing situation, consider driving your child to and from school. You might also find some of your neighbors will be interested in carpooling with you.

CHECKLIST

- ✓ Schedule to meet the bus driver
- ✓ Go over allergy action plan and fill out any required forms
- ✓ Discuss the bus rules and policies
- ✓ Will the bus be used for other events?
- ✓ Will your child have an assigned seat that's frequently cleaned?
- ✓ How and when will they receive training?
- ✓ Where will the epinephrine be located?
- ✓ How will substitute drivers be informed and trained?
- ✓ What's the route and how many buses will your child ride each day?
- ✓ If you don't feel comfortable, consider other options

NOTES

Chapter 8

Talking to Teachers

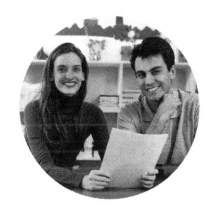

It's critical that the teacher fully understands your child's allergy; they'll be one of the biggest team members to help keep your child safe. Have a heart-to-heart with them and let them know how you feel. Also, let them know how much you need and truly appreciate their help.

Discuss with them how the school day runs and ask them what areas they believe might be a concern. They know the daily flow of the school and classroom, and will know more about any potential problems that might need to be addressed.

Go over your child's allergy action plan together. Make sure they fully understand the signs and symptoms of an allergic reaction, and know how to administer an epinephrine auto-injector. Talk to them and find out how comfortable they are with the situation. Again, be sure to share stories, pictures, anything to help them "get it".

Offer to provide materials

Let them know you want to help them in any way you can. If they're writing and sending a letter to the parents, offer them assistance in writing it if needed.

Discuss how the allergy will be brought up to the other students. Kids are usually very supportive and protective of their classmates, if they understand the allergy. Offer to share books, videos, or any other materials that will help them and your child's classmates gain a better understanding of food allergies.

Also, discuss reminding the parents often about the food allergy, especially after holiday breaks. They could easily state a reminder in a newsletter or other source saying, "Thank you for helping keep your child's classmate safe by...." and then list the food allergy safety rules.

Classroom snacks and parties

Find out if it's possible to have no food in the classroom during the first few weeks, when everything is getting adjusted. Are classroom snacks their decision or does the principal have the final word? Discuss the possibility of not having snacks in the classroom during the year and only using non-food items for parties, celebrations, and rewards. Another possibility you could discuss is only allowing "safe" snacks that are individually wrapped and labeled.

You might want to offer to make a safe treat for the entire class during parties and celebrations. But, be sure to consider your time and finances, and don't try to do things that are too difficult for you. You have enough things going on and don't need to create additional stress for yourself. It's NOT your responsibility to bake or provide items for the whole class.

Also, if there are other children who have food allergies or intolerances to different foods, baking may become more difficult. Be sure to find out what items you'll need to avoid, because as you already know....excluding any child from a celebration is unfair and heartbreaking.

Discuss the possibility of parties being held less often during the school year. Make sure they know how much advance notice you'll need of any classroom parties and school celebrations.

Try to participate in class parties as much as possible. If food is being ordered for a party, ask if you can have a part in helping decide where they will order the food from or what they will purchase. Consider going in before the party starts so you'll have time to read the labels and check any items that will be served.

Limiting parties may actually be a welcomed idea to teachers, because parties take away from learning and their normal routine. Standardized testing has teachers needing to teach more content in a shorter time frame.

Safe Snacks

Can you help them compile a list of resources and ideas on allergy-friendly snacks and non-food party items? This might be very helpful to give to the other parents. Be sure the list includes a warning: Ingredients and manufacturing processes often change, ALWAYS read the label before purchasing.

Also, provide a container with safe snacks for your child so they're never left out of receiving a classroom treat. Let your child pick out items they love, but maybe don't get to enjoy often at home. That way, they'll look forward to getting their treat. Make sure the teacher keeps the container in a safe place in the classroom. Consider using items that have a longer shelf life, like fruit snacks or individually packaged pretzels.

Let the teacher know they'll need to watch out for children trying to share or trade their food, drinks, napkins and utensils. Discuss why your child shouldn't use the public drinking fountain and should have access to a marked water bottle or cup.

Label reading and cross-contact

Educate them on label reading and give them a list of different names for the allergen. Inform them that certain allergens can be found in many products like art supplies, pet food (if there's a classroom pet), soaps and lotions.

If it has a label, they need to read it! If the items are already in the classroom, ask to see them and go over the labels. You can find a list of sites that provide label reading information in our resource section.

Discuss cross-contact (contamination from the allergen) and properly cleaning the allergen from surfaces. This is especially important if the classroom is used for after school events. Can the custodian pay special attention to cleaning areas like desks, floors, doorknobs, etc. in your child's classroom?

The allergen could get transferred to books, computers, etc. Discuss having your child assigned their own set of classroom books, supplies and manipulatives for the school year. Ask if they can frequently clean the computer keyboards and have a specific computer that remains free from the allergen. Make sure they don't use candy for manipulatives for math, bingo or other activities.

Washing hands

Your child needs to wash their hands before and after eating. Discuss with the teacher how this can be achieved. Having all the students wash their hands after lunch should be discussed with the teacher. Request your child is first in line and have them use a paper towel to turn on and off the handle. Oftentimes, kindergarten classes have a bathroom or sink in their classroom, which makes this process easier.

Find out if they can have all the students in the classroom wash their hands as soon as they get to school in the morning. A great benefit to that is it will also cut down on spreading germs and sickness. Is there a way to ask guests who had the allergen, to wash their hands before entering the classroom?

Certain days or activities might not allow students to wash their hands, and using wet wipes might be a good backup to have in the classroom. Let them know: Hand sanitizer removes germs, it DOESN'T remove the allergen.

Bullying and Exclusion

Find out what will happen if a student bullies or teases your child about their food allergy. Discuss the seriousness of bullying and ask the teacher if they can pay attention to what the students are saying and doing. One thing about working with younger children is they often tattle on each other.

Also discuss that isolation and exclusion of activities is truly unfair to your child just because they have an allergy. ALL children want to be included, and having a life-threatening allergy is not something they chose. The stress of being excluded from the activity, along with fearing possible contamination, is awful to put a child through.

Specials (art, music, gym)

Other teachers you'll want to talk to are the art, music, and gym teachers. Make sure the art teacher is trained on label reading and reads the labels for all art supplies. Craft items may contain traces of the allergens.

In music class, do the children get their own instrument? If not, see if one can be specifically assigned to your child. A child may have music class right after they consume the allergen at lunch and could contaminate the instrument.

If the cafeteria and gym class share the same area, has the floor been cleaned after meals? Many times kids can go play until lunch is over, but they haven't washed their hands. Are there ways to help decrease the possibility of allergens being transferring onto playground or sporting equipment?

Thank You's

Remember - teachers have good intentions and a desire to help others, that's most likely why they're in the profession. Unfortunately, sometimes people forget or have multiple tasks and things get overlooked. Make sure you and your child stand out in their mind.

A good way to remind them is by sending them a thank you card. In it, you can list the ways they help make sure your child is safe and how much you appreciate it. Not only is this helpful in reminding them about safety for your child, it would mean a lot to them to hear how thankful you are, for all that they do.

Don't assume telling them once will be sufficient. Remind them about food allergy safety, and thank them throughout the year!

CHECKLIST

- ✓ Go over action plan and administering epinephrine
- ✓ Have a heart-to-heart conversation and share your concerns
- ✓ Offer to supply books, videos or any other materials you may have
- ✓ Who will write letters and how will they inform the classmates?
- ✓ Discuss "no food" or limited food in the classroom
- ✓ If you have the time and finances, offer to bake treats for parties
- ✓ Request advanced notice of parties and field trips
- ✓ Offer to provide safe snack ideas and non-food reward ideas
- ✓ Provide safe snacks to be kept in the classroom for your child
- ✓ Have them watch out for children sharing or trading items
- ✓ Discuss label reading with all your child's teachers
- ✓ Discuss cross-contact and cleaning surfaces

- ✓ Request your child's assigned their own set of books and supplies
- ✓ Discuss hand washing before and after eating
- ✓ Discuss notifying classroom guests about the allergy
- ✓ Discuss classroom rules and bullying
- ✓ Discuss isolation from activities
- ✓ Meet with the art, music, and gym teachers to discuss safety
- ✓ Continually remind them of allergy safety tips throughout the year
- ✓ Send thank you cards to let them know they are appreciated

NOTES

Chapter 9

Helping Your Child Prepare

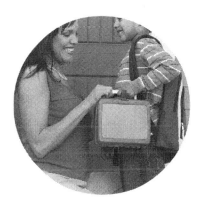

Besides meeting with the school, you'll also have to help your child get prepared. One of the biggest things to remember: what comes OUT of your mouth can greatly effect what goes INTO their mouth.

Teach allergy safety to your child and remind them often! Role-play different scenarios with your child to help them prepare to handle different situations they might encounter. You can pretend you're a friend trying to offer them a snack or other potential scenarios they might face.

Children often believe that the adult or classmate offering them a treat understands food allergy safety and would never do anything to hurt them. Discuss with them how some people don't understand or that they make mistakes.

Teaching Self-Advocacy

Start teaching them to self-advocate. Politely say, "No thank you, I have a food allergy" when they're offered food that may be unsafe. Make sure they know they MUST have all foods given to them checked, and also what adults they can have read the labels for them.

Teach your child the signs and symptoms of an allergic reaction, and what they need to do in an emergency. Describe different symptoms they could feel in an allergic reaction. Show pictures of changes they may see on their skin. Again, role play different situations and discuss what they will do, who they will tell, etc.

In elementary, they can't always tell what items contain the allergen. They don't fully understand cross-contact and surely can't read all those confusing ingredients on the labels. Make sure others understand this and know how important it is, that they help look out for your child's safety.

Always teach your child to recognize the allergen. Find pictures on the Internet, in books, and at the store. What does it look like and how does it look in different forms? If it's a nut allergy, make sure they know the different nuts and what they look like in and out of their shell. What do nuts look like chopped up in cookies?

Start teaching them about label reading as soon as possible. Show them where the allergy information is listed on a product. Take them to the grocery store and show them different products that are safe and unsafe and let them know why. Make sure they understand products can change and become unsafe, and need to be checked EVERY time.

Teach your child how to use an epinephrine auto-injector when age-appropriate. Don't expect them to use it in an emergency, but help them be able to communicate about it if needed. Make sure they know why they must have it at all times. Establish rules on how they can't play with it, and always need to keep it with them. Help them find a holder they'll like to carry, maybe a specific color or pattern.

If they feel they're being bullied or teased, discuss what they should do and whom they should tell. Role-play how they can handle this type of situation. Emphasize how a real friend will never make them do something they shouldn't do. Discuss peer pressure and how sometimes they may have to do things alone.

Make sure they've been introduced to the guidance counselor, nurse and principal, and actually feel comfortable around them. It's one thing to say, "you can trust this person", but you need to know if they actually will.

Discuss when they should go to the guidance counselor, nurse, or principal for help... feeling bullied, etc.

Always listen to what they're saying; they'll give clues to how they're feeling and what's going on around them. How do they talk to their toys or other people? Do they talk about feeling "left out", do they act anxious, etc.?

Providing Items

Provide different forms of materials to teach about food allergy safety for your child and others. People have different ways they learn best (like visual, audio and hands-on) and using different forms of materials and activities can help them better understand.

Provide safe snacks they'll look forward to eating and make sure they have plenty of safe snacks at school. Bake and freeze items to have ready for a "party emergency". Make cookies, brownies, or bake cupcakes - then freeze. This will help you be prepared to send baked treats in just minutes.

Provide a medical bracelet or piece of jewelry that can easily let others know of your child's allergy. If your child will wear a bracelet, help them find one they'll enjoy wearing each day. Make sure it's one that clearly shows others about the allergy and not just a "cool" one that might be easily mistaken for a novelty or regular bracelet. Younger children can also wear an allergy alert tag on their shoelaces.

If they play sports or are very active, you may want to consider using a second form of awareness, like temporary tattoos, shirts, or other items. Then, they'll have a backup if they accidentally lose or break their bracelet. This could also give them multiple ways of informing/reminding others about their allergy during the first couple of weeks. You can find food allergy alert tattoos at www.allergyfreezone.com.

Always go with your gut. If you don't feel comfortable with a situation, avoid it. Be creative and think outside the box. If your child doesn't go on the field trip, let them help plan something else they can do instead. If they were unable to eat the cupcake at school...consider baking some together that the whole family can enjoy.

CHECKLIST

- ✓ Teaching names of the allergen and how it looks in different forms
- ✓ Teaching how to read labels – show and discuss items when at store
- ✓ Reminding them not to eat anything that hasn't been approved
- ✓ Teaching them who can check if the food is safe and read labels
- ✓ Saying, "No thank you, I have a food allergy" to unapproved foods
- ✓ Washing hands before and after eating
- ✓ Watching the environment to help avoid going near the allergen
- ✓ Not to share or trade food, drinks, napkins or utensils
- ✓ Teaching how things are cross-contaminated
- ✓ Making sure they know the signs and symptoms of a reaction
- ✓ Knowing what to do if they experience a reaction

- ✓ Knowing how to administer epinephrine when appropriate
- ✓ Providing safe snacks they'll look forward to eating
- ✓ Baking and freezing goods to have for a "party emergency"
- ✓ Providing allergy awareness items for your child to use/wear
- ✓ Teaching them how to handle bullying and teasing
- ✓ Reminding your child to carry medication at all times
- ✓ Teaching them self-advocacy skills
- ✓ Encouraging your child and building self-esteem
- ✓ Consider finding parents or groups where your child can play
- ✓ Role play different scenarios with your child and others
- ✓ Providing materials to teach about food allergy safety
- ✓ Frequently communicating with school, especially the nurse and teachers
- ✓ Participate in all meetings/conferences concerning your child

NOTES

Chapter 10

Food Allergies in the News

Here are some stories that have been in the media, you might want to discuss during your team meeting. I do warn you that some of the children had a fatal reaction from their food allergy, and it's very heartbreaking to read.

These stories are not meant to scare you, but make you aware of things that have happened. It's so important to share these stories to help make sure it doesn't happen to another child again.

Thankfully, people are starting to understand how serious food allergies are, but we still have so many that need to be educated. When someone doesn't take food allergies seriously, sharing these just might help them "get it".

Field Trips

A 9-year-old had a known peanut allergy, but the school's sack lunches that were provided had items containing peanuts. After tasting a cookie, he reported not feeling well and waited on the bus while his class continued with the field trip. His condition worsened and they administered an epinephrine injection, but it was too late.

Full story:
http://abcnews.go.com/Health/AllergiesNews/story?id=4856211&page=1

His mother was one of the speakers that addressed the Senate about the need for guidelines at school for children with food allergies.

Years after being introduced, the Food Allergy & Anaphylaxis Management Act (FAAMA) went into effect in 2011, and in 2013, the CDC released national guidelines.

Read more about FAAMA at:
http://www.foodallergy.org/laws-and-regulations/faama

Cafeteria

A **13-year-old** ordered French fries from the school cafeteria, but dairy protein was on the tongs that were used to serve her food. She thought she was having an asthma attack and went to the school office. A teacher quickly tried to retrieve the epinephrine out of her locker, but she had gone into cardiac arrest before it could be administered.

Full article:
http://allergicliving.com/index.php/2010/07/02/sabrinas-law-the-girl-and-the-allergy-law/

Her mother helped advocate, and in 2006, "Sabrina's Law" went into effect in Ontario. This helped set up anaphylaxis and allergy guidelines for Ontario schools, and later contributed to the development of laws and policies in the United States.

Read more about Sabrina's Law at:

http://foodallergycanada.ca/resources/sabrinas-law/

Classroom

A mother had checked the snacks that were going to be given during the classroom party, yet she received a phone call that her **7-year-old** son had taken a bite of a peanut butter granola bar. He was given liquid antihistamine and didn't appear to have symptoms at that time, but then experienced a delayed reaction. At the hospital they had to perform CPR and put him on a life support machine. Thankfully, he was able to return home days later.

Full story:
http://www.ketv.com/Boy-Survives-Delayed-Reaction-To-Peanut-Allergy/-/9675214/11671584/-/item/0/-/11b3hx5z/-/index.html

A 13-year old had a fatal reaction after eating Chinese food that was ordered for a class celebration. According to the article, the teacher had called the restaurant multiple times to check that the food would be free from the allergen.

Full article:
http://allergicliving.com/2010/12/20/anaphylaxis-tragedy-for-chicago-teen/

In 2011, Illinois became the first state to have a "stock" epinephrine law.

Playground/Recess

A classmate shared a food item with a **7-year old** girl on the playground. She informed a teacher when she started having symptoms, but there wasn't an epinephrine auto-injector for her at the school. By the time the EMS arrived, she had already gone into cardiac arrest.

Full story:
http://abcnews.go.com/Health/AllergiesFood/allergic-girl-died-school-peanut-child/story?id=15341841#.UBXxP2ht2FI

Her mother helped advocate for getting epinephrine stocked for any child to use in an emergency, and in 2012, "Amarria's Law" went in effect in Virginia.

In 2013, President Obama signed into law the School Access to Emergency Epinephrine Act.

Visit FARE for more information on school epinephrine legislation & guidelines in the U.S.:
http://www.foodallergy.org/advocacy/epinephrine/map

Bus

An American Red Cross Chapter in Massachusetts gave their Hometown Heroes Award to a bus driver and high school senior for helping a student that was having a severe allergic reaction. The student didn't have her epinephrine, so the senior shared her auto-injector and the driver quickly administered it.

Full story:

http://www.masslive.com/news/index.ssf/2015/03/agawam_bus_driver_high_school.html

How You Can Help

- Keep these families in your thoughts and prayers. Even though some of these stories are several years old, the pain from their loss will always be there.

- Share their stories to educate others and help prevent another child from being placed in the same situation.

- Help change laws to increase safety for those with life-threatening food allergies. Visit FARE for ways that you can become involved:
  http://www.foodallergy.org/advocacy2

Thank You No Nuts Moms Group - Many of these stories were found in their post "Remembering Those We Have Lost To Food Allergies".
http://nonutsmomsgroup.weebly.com/1/post/2012/02/remembering-those-we-have-lost-to-food-allergies.html

Helpful Resources

Visit www.allergyfreezone.com/resources for downloadable checklists & food allergy resources.

Books

Parents

- *How to Manage Your Child's Life-Threatening Food Allergies: Practical Tips for Everyday Life* by Linda Marienhoff Coss
- *The Food Allergy Experience* by Dr. Ruchi Gupta
- *Understanding and Managing your Child's Food Allergies* by Dr. Scott Sicherer
- *One Of The Gang* by Gina Clowes

Kids

- *The Princess and the Peanut: A Royally Allergic Tale* by Sue Ganz-Schmitt and Micah Chambers-Goldberg
- *Allie the Allergic Elephant* (series) by Nicole Smith
- *The Bugabees: Friends With Food Allergies* (series) by Amy Recob
- *HumFree the Bee Has a Food Allergy by Alison Grace Johansen*
- Alexander Storybook Series – available through FARE

Products

Food Allergy Awareness Items - Stickers, Tattoos, Lunch Bags, Signs, and more! www.allergyfreezone.com

Magazines

Allergic Living - http://www.allergicliving.com
Gluten Free & More - http://www.glutenfreeandmore.com

Audio/Video

Parents

- KFA's webinars:
  http://community.kidswithfoodallergies.org/pages/webinars

- FARE's webinars: https://www.foodallergy.org/tools-and-resources/webinars

- Discovery Channel's *An Emerging Epidemic: Food Allergies in America*: http://www.foodallergy.org/emerging-epidemic#.VSrAeEv4QpE

- Food Allergy Canada videos & presentations:
  http://foodallergycanada.ca/resources/videos-presentations/

Kids

- *Food Allergies Rock!* by Kyle Dine http://www.kyledine.com

- *The Allergy Song* by The Wiggles
  http://www.youtube.com/watch?v=iAs4lZkK8mY

- *Arthur: Binky Goes Nuts* (DVD)
  http://shop.pbskids.org/binky-goes-nuts-dvd.html

Allergy & Asthma Information in U.S. & Canada

- Food Allergy & Anaphylaxis Connection Team (FAACT) - http://www.foodallergyawareness.org

- Food Allergy Research & Education (FARE) - http://www.foodallergy.org

- Kids With Food Allergies (KFA) - http://www.kidswithfoodallergies.org

- Allergy Kids - http://www.allergykids.com

- The Allergy and Asthma Network - Mothers of Asthmatics - http://www.aanma.org

- Asthma and Allergy Foundation of America - http://www.aafa.org

- American Academy of Allergy, Asthma & Immunology - http://www.aaaai.org

- Food Allergy Canada – http://www.foodallergycanada.ca

- Allergy/Asthma Information Association – http://www.aaia.ca

- Health Canada – http://www.hc-sc.gc.ca

- CSACI (Canadian Society of Allergy & Clinical Immunology) - www.csaci.ca

- CAAIF (Canadian Allergy, Asthma & Immunology Foundation) – http://www.allergyfoundation.ca

Information for Schools

FAME Food Allergy Management and Education Program
http://www.stlouischildrens.org/health-resources/advocacy-outreach/food-allergy-management-and-education

CDC "Voluntary Guidelines for Managing Food Allergies In Schools and Early Care and Education Programs "
http://www.cdc.gov/healthyyouth/foodallergies

FAACT's "FAACTs for Schools Program"
http://www.foodallergyawareness.org/education/faacts_for_schools_program-15/

FARE's "Food Allergies: Keeping Students Safe and Included"
http://www.foodallergy.org/education-network

National School Board Association – "Safe at School and Ready to Learn: A Comprehensive Policy Guide for Protecting Students with Life-threatening Food Allergies" http://www.nsba.org/safe-school-and-ready-learn-comprehensive-policy-guide-protecting-students-life-threatening-food

"Addressing Food Allergies in Schools" Powerpoint from NSBA -
http://www.nsba.org/addressing-food-allergies-schools-powerpoint-presentation

"Managing Food Allergies in School – What School Staff Needs to Know" (video/slideshow) from AllergyHome
http://www.allergyhome.org/schools/management-of-food-allergies-in-school-what-school-staff-need-to-know

"How to C.A.R.E. for Students with Food Allergies: What Educators Should Know" (online training) from AllergyReady.com
http://allergyready.com

Cafeteria

School Nutrition Association – Food Allergy Resources
podcasts/webinars: http://www.schoolnutrition.org

Nurses

Food Allergy Toolkit for School Nurses
www.nasn.org/ToolsResources/FoodAllergyandAnaphylaxis

EpiPen4Schools® from Mylan: https://www.epipen4schools.com

Teachers
Activities for Students

- FAACT's Food Allergy School Curricula Program - http://www.foodallergyawareness.org/education/school_cu rricula_program-2/

- Kyle Dine & Friends Food Allergy Awareness Videos - http://www.foodallergyvideo.com

- Coloring Pages - http://arizonafoodallergy.org/coloring-pages.html

- Lesson Plan for *Binky Goes Nuts* - http://www.pbs.org/parents/arthur/lesson/health/

- Be a PAL: Protect A Life™ From Food Allergies by FARE - http://www.foodallergy.org/be-a-pal

- Games & Coloring Pages - http://www.aaaai.org/conditions-and-treatments/just-for-kids.aspx

- A list of Non-Food Rewards - http://community.kidswithfoodallergies.org/blog/non-food-rewards-for-children-with-food-allergies-new-handout

- Allergy-Friendly "Fun" Ideas - http://pinterest.com/allergyfreezone

Cross-Contact
- FAACT - How To Prevent Cross-Contact and Accidental Environmental Exposure: http://www.foodallergyawareness.org/foodallergy/cross-contact-15/

- FARE – Avoiding Cross-Contact http://www.foodallergy.org/tools-and-resources/managing-food-allergies/cross-contact

Label Reading
- FAACT - http://www.foodallergyawareness.org/foodallergy/food_labeling-10/food_labels-50/

- KFA - http://www.kidswithfoodallergies.org/page/choosing-safe-foods.aspx

- FARE - http://www.foodallergy.org/food-labels

Lunch/Snack Ideas
- Allergy Free Zone's Pinterest page for allergy-friendly ideas: www.pinterest.com/allergyfreezone

Crafts

- KFA's list of "Potential Food Allergens in Preschool, School, Camp Crafts & Activities": http://www.kidswithfoodallergies.org/page/potential-food-allergens-in-preschool-school-camp-crafts-activities.aspx

Bullying

FAACT's Information on Bullying
http://www.foodallergyawareness.org/education/bullying-16/

FARE's "Food Allergy Bullying: It's Not a Joke"
http://www.foodallergy.org/its-not-a-joke#.V5VIEFfbjEw

Stopbullying.gov "Bullying and Youth with Disabilities and Special Health Needs" http://www.stopbullying.gov/at-risk/groups/special-needs/

Food Allergy Action Plans

- Food Allergy & Anaphylaxis Emergency Care Plan www.foodallergy.org/faap

- AAAAI Anaphylaxis Emergency Action Plan http://www.aaaai.org/Aaaai/media/MediaLibrary/PDF%20Documents/Libraries/Anaphylaxis-Emergency-Action-Plan.pdf

504

FAACT's Civil Rights Advocacy section has information on 504s and accommodations.
http://www.foodallergyawareness.org/civil-rights-advocacy/

Wrightslaw.com has articles, legal references, cases and settlements that deal with allergies, anaphylaxis, 504s, and ADA.
http://www.wrightslaw.com/info/allergy.index.htm

U.S. Department of Education:
http://www2.ed.gov/about/offices/list/ocr/504faq.html

"Section 504 and Written Management Plans" by FARE
http://www.foodallergy.org/advocacy/disability

"Sample Section 504 Plans for Managing Food Allergies" by KFA:
http://www.kidswithfoodallergies.org/page/sample-section-504-plan-for-food-allergy.aspx

Support Groups/Playgroups

FAACT-
http://www.foodallergyawareness.org/education/support_group_d
evelopment-5/food_allergy_support_groups-13/

Kid's With Food Allergies-
http://www.kidswithfoodallergies.org/groups.php

No Nuts Mom's Group -
http://nonutsmomsgroup.weebly.com/groups.html

FARE- http://www.foodallergy.org/support-groups

Anaphylaxis Canada -
http://www.anaphylaxis.ca/en/i_want/resources/support_groups.h
tml

Disclaimer

The resources listed in this book are provided for informational
purposes only. They are intended to be used as a guide when
working with your allergist and team members. Neither the author
nor Allergy Free Zone, LLC is responsible for the content of these
resources, sites or organizations. Any information found should not
replace professional medical or legal advice. Be sure to discuss any
questions of a medical nature with your physician, and legal
questions with your attorney.

NOTES

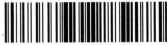
Made in the USA
Middletown, DE
30 August 2016